Celiac Disease

Cookbook for Seniors

Nutritious and Tasty Gluten-Free Recipes to Enhance Older individuals Lifestyle

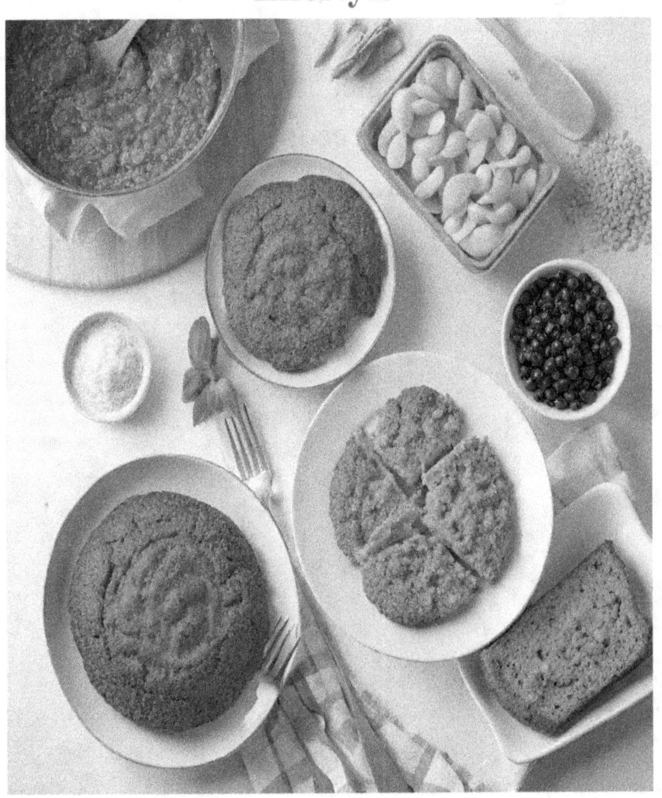

Dr. Tate Mandara

Table Of Contents

INTRODUCTION

Meet Catherine, a vibrant senior who rediscovered joy in her meals with the "Celiac Disease Cookbook for Seniors." Struggling with the limitations of her Celiac diagnosis, Catherine felt the weight of bland and restrictive meals. As she delved into the cookbook, a culinary transformation unfolded. Breakfasts turned into a celebration with nutty millet breakfast bowl and banana oat pancakes that didn't compromise on flavor. Lunch became a flavorful adventure with salmon avocado lettuce wraps and watermelon poke bowls. For dinner, she relished zucchini lasagna and gluten-free chicken alfredo, savoring every bite without worry. The sides section introduced her to garlic roasted Brussels sprouts and mashed sweet potatoes, enhancing her meals with delightful textures and tastes. Snack time became a joy with string cheese and raisins delights.

Even soups and stews found a place in her heart, warming her soul with options like creamy carrot ginger soup. The Fish & Seafood chapter became a weekly ritual, from balsamic glazed salmon to grilled halibut with mango salsa. Dessert, once a distant dream, became a reality with flourless chocolate avocado brownies and strawberry lemonade angel pie. Catherine's journey proves that age is no barrier to savoring life, one delicious and gluten-free meal at a time. This cookbook became her culinary companion, turning each meal into a celebration of flavor and well-being.

CHAPTER ONE

What is Celiac Disease?

Celiac Disease is an autoimmune disorder triggered by the ingestion of gluten, a protein found in wheat, barley, and rye. When individuals with Celiac Disease consume gluten, their immune system mistakenly attacks the small intestine, damaging its lining and hindering nutrient absorption. This chronic condition can manifest at any age and often leads to various symptoms, including abdominal pain, diarrhea, fatigue, and weight loss. The hallmark of Celiac Disease is the presence of specific antibodies and genetic markers. Diagnosis involves blood tests and, if indicated, an intestinal biopsy. All you can do is avoid gluten for the rest of your life.

By avoiding gluten-containing foods, individuals with Celiac Disease can alleviate symptoms, promote intestinal healing, and prevent complications. Awareness of Celiac Disease is crucial, as it often goes undiagnosed, and timely intervention can significantly improve the quality of life for those affected.

Common Symptoms in Seniors

Seniors with Celiac Disease may experience a range of symptoms that differ from those seen in younger individuals. Common symptoms in seniors include unexplained weight loss, fatigue, and nutritional deficiencies, as the damaged intestinal lining hinders proper nutrient absorption. Gastrointestinal issues such as chronic diarrhea, abdominal pain, and bloating are prevalent but may be subtle.

Seniors might also encounter mood changes, cognitive difficulties, or neuropathy due to nutrient deficiencies.

It's crucial to note that Celiac symptoms can vary widely, and some seniors may be asymptomatic. As Celiac Disease can mimic age-related conditions, diagnosing it in seniors can be challenging. A high level of awareness among healthcare professionals is essential to identify and address Celiac Disease promptly in older individuals, improving their overall health and well-being.

Diagnosis and Treatment

Diagnosing and treating Celiac Disease in seniors involves a multifaceted approach.

Diagnosis often begins with blood tests to detect specific antibodies, followed by confirmation through an intestinal biopsy. Given that Celiac symptoms can mimic other age-related conditions, a high level of clinical suspicion is crucial for timely diagnosis in seniors. Once diagnosed, the primary and only effective treatment is a strict and lifelong gluten-free diet. Seniors with Celiac Disease must diligently avoid gluten-containing foods to alleviate symptoms and prevent complications. Additionally, nutritional support may be necessary to address deficiencies caused by malabsorption.

Collaborative efforts between healthcare professionals, including dietitians, gastroenterologists, and primary care physicians, play a vital role in managing Celiac Disease in seniors, ensuring optimal care, and enhancing their overall quality of life.

Managing Celiac Disease in Later Years

Managing Celiac Disease in later years requires a holistic approach to address the unique needs of seniors. Adopting a strict gluten-free diet is the cornerstone of management, involving the elimination of wheat, barley, and rye from their meals. Seniors should collaborate closely with healthcare professionals, including dietitians, to ensure nutritional adequacy and monitor for potential deficiencies resulting from malabsorption.

Regular medical follow-ups and screenings are essential to assess intestinal healing and address any emerging health concerns.

Beyond dietary modifications, managing Celiac Disease in seniors involves fostering a supportive environment, enhancing awareness among caregivers, and providing resources for navigating social situations that involve food. With a comprehensive strategy, seniors can effectively navigate the challenges of Celiac Disease, maintain their well-being, and enjoy a fulfilling, gluten-free lifestyle in their later years.

Foods to Eat and Avoid

Seniors with Celiac Disease benefit from a meticulous understanding of foods to embrace and avoid to maintain optimal health. Foods rich in naturally gluten-free grains like rice, quinoa, and corn, along with fresh fruits, vegetables, and lean proteins, form the foundation of a Celiac-friendly diet. Seniors should opt for certified gluten-free alternatives for staples like bread and pasta. However, they must steer clear of wheat, barley, and rye, found in various processed foods and condiments.

Reading labels becomes crucial to identifying hidden gluten sources. Additionally, seniors should be cautious with oats, ensuring they are labeled as gluten-free due to potential cross-contamination. A balanced and varied diet, supplemented with gluten-free grains and fortified foods, aids seniors in managing Celiac Disease effectively, promoting digestive health and overall well-being.

Tips for cooking and preparing Celiac-friendly meals

Cooking and preparing Celiac-friendly meals involves creativity and attention to detail to ensure a delicious and safe dining experience. Begin by establishing a gluten-free kitchen, designating specific utensils, cutting boards, and cookware to avoid cross-contamination.

Embrace naturally gluten-free grains like rice, quinoa, and millet, and explore gluten-free flours for baking. Read labels diligently, even for seemingly unrelated products, to identify hidden gluten sources. Experiment with alternative flours and starches like almond flour, coconut flour, and tapioca starch to diversify your recipes. Opt for fresh, whole foods, and prioritize naturally gluten-free ingredients to enhance nutritional value.

Engage in meal planning, preparing large batches that can be frozen for convenience. Finally, stay informed about gluten-free substitutions and be open to discovering new and flavorful gluten-free recipes to enjoy a varied and satisfying Celiac-friendly culinary journey.

CHAPTER TWO

BREAKFAST RECIPES

Banana Oat Pancakes

Serving: One

Ingredients:
- 1 ripe banana
- 1/2 cup gluten-free oats
- 1/2 teaspoon baking powder
- 1/4 teaspoon cinnamon
- 1/4 cup milk (dairy or non-dairy)
- 1 large egg

Instructions:

1. In a blender, combine the banana, oats, baking powder, cinnamon, milk, and egg. Blend until smooth.

2. Heat a non-stick skillet over medium heat and lightly grease with oil or butter.

3. Pour 1/4 cup of batter onto the skillet for each pancake.

4. Cook until bubbles form on the surface, then flip and cook until golden brown.

5. Serve with fresh fruit or maple syrup.

Nutritional Value:

Calories: 280

Carbohydrates: 45g

Protein: 9g

Fat: 7g

Fiber: 6g

Sodium: 300mg

Creamy Polenta with Chorizo

Serving: One

Ingredients:
- 1/2 cup polenta
- 2 cups water
- 1/4 teaspoon salt
- 2 ounces gluten-free chorizo, sliced

Instructions:

1. In a saucepan, bring the water to a boil. Gradually whisk in the polenta and salt.

2. Reduce the heat to low and cook, stirring frequently, for 15-20 minutes until creamy.

3. In a separate skillet, cook the chorizo slices until browned.

4. Serve the creamy polenta topped with the cooked chorizo.

Nutritional Value:

Calories: 320

Carbohydrates: 30g

Protein: 12g

Fat: 15g

Fiber: 3g

Sodium: 600mg

Biscuits and Gravy

Serving: One

Ingredients:
- 1 gluten-free biscuit
- 2 gluten-free sausage patties
- 1 cup gluten-free gravy

Instructions:

1. Prepare the gluten-free biscuits and sausage patties according to package instructions.

2. Warm the gluten-free gravy in a saucepan over medium heat.

3. Split the biscuit in half, place the sausage patty on each half, and pour the warm gravy over the top.

Nutritional Value:

Calories: 450

Carbohydrates: 35g

Protein: 18g

Fat: 25g

Fiber: 2g

Sodium: 800mg

Rhubarb Muffins

Serving: One

Ingredients:

- 1 cup gluten-free flour
- 1/2 cup almond flour
- 1/2 cup sugar
- 1 teaspoon baking powder
- 1/2 teaspoon baking soda
- 1/4 teaspoon salt
- 1/2 cup yogurt (dairy or non-dairy)
- 1/4 cup oil
- 1 teaspoon vanilla extract
- 1 cup chopped rhubarb

Instructions:

1. Preheat the oven to 375°F (190°C) and line a muffin tin with paper liners.

2. In a bowl, whisk together the gluten-free flour, almond flour, sugar, baking powder, baking soda, and salt.

3. In another bowl, mix the yogurt, oil, and vanilla extract.

4. Combine the wet and dry ingredients, then fold in the chopped rhubarb.

5. Divide the batter among the muffin cups and bake for 20-25 minutes or until a toothpick inserted comes out clean.

Nutritional Value:
Calories: 180
Carbohydrates: 25g
Protein: 4g
Fat: 8g
Fiber: 2g
Sodium: 200mg

Cinnamon Quinoa Bake

Serving: One

Ingredients:

•1/2 cup quinoa

•1 cup milk (dairy or non-dairy)

•1/4 cup maple syrup

•1/2 teaspoon cinnamon

•1/4 cup chopped nuts (e.g., almonds, walnuts)

Instructions:

1. Preheat the oven to 375°F (190°C) and lightly grease a baking dish.

2. Rinse the quinoa and place it in the baking dish.

3. In a bowl, whisk together the milk, maple syrup, and cinnamon. Pour over the quinoa.

4. Cover the dish with foil and bake for 30 minutes.

5. Remove the foil, sprinkle the chopped nuts on top, and bake for an additional 15 minutes.

Nutritional Value:

Calories: 280

Carbohydrates: 40g

Protein: 8g

Fat: 10g

Fiber: 4g

Sodium: 100mg

Tomato Tart

Serving: One

Ingredients:

•1 gluten-free pie crust

•1 cup cherry tomatoes, halved

•1/4 cup shredded mozzarella cheese

•2 tablespoons chopped fresh basil

•Salt and pepper to taste

Instructions:

1. Preheat the oven to 375°F (190°C).
2. Place the gluten-free pie crust on a baking sheet.

3. Arrange the halved cherry tomatoes on the crust, then sprinkle with mozzarella cheese and chopped basil.

4. Season with salt and pepper.

5. Bake for 25-30 minutes or until the crust is golden and the tomatoes are softened.

Nutritional Value:

Calories: 220

Carbohydrates: 20g

Protein: 5g

Fat: 12g

Fiber: 2g

Sodium: 300mg

Nutty Millet Breakfast Bowl

Serving: One

Ingredients:
- 1/2 cup cooked millet
- 1/4 cup chopped mixed nuts (e.g., almonds, pecans, walnuts)
- 1/4 cup fresh berries (e.g., strawberries, blueberries)
- 1 tablespoon honey or maple syrup

Instructions:

1. In a bowl, combine the cooked millet, chopped mixed nuts, and fresh berries.

2. Drizzle with honey or maple syrup.

3. Serve warm or cold.

Nutritional Value:

Calories: 280

Carbohydrates: 35g

Protein: 6g

Fat: 14g

Fiber: 5g

Sodium: 10mg

Gluten-Free Pancakes

Serving: One

Ingredients:

- 1/2 cup gluten-free flour
- 1 tablespoon sugar
- 1/2 teaspoon baking powder
- 1/4 teaspoon salt
- 1/2 cup milk (dairy or non-dairy)
- 1 large egg
- 1 tablespoon melted butter or oil
- 1/2 teaspoon vanilla extract

Instructions:

1. In a bowl, whisk together the gluten-free flour, sugar, baking powder, and salt.

2. In another bowl, whisk the milk, egg, melted butter or oil, and vanilla extract.

3. Pour the wet ingredients into the dry ingredients and stir until just combined.

4. Grease a non-stick skillet with butter or oil and heat it over medium heat.

5. For each pancake, add 1/4 cup of batter to the skillet.

6. Cook until surface bubbles appear, then turn and continue cooking until golden brown.

7. Serve with your favorite toppings such as fresh fruit, maple syrup, or yogurt.

Nutritional Value:

Calories: 250

Carbohydrates: 35g

Protein: 6g

Fat: 9g

Fiber: 2g

Sodium: 400mg

CHAPTER THREE

LUNCH RECIPES

Grilled Chicken over Greens with Lemon Vinaigrette

Serving: One

Cooking Time: 15 minutes

Ingredients:

•4 oz grilled chicken breast

•2 cups mixed greens

•1/4 cup chopped red onion

•1/4 cup chopped bell peppers

•1/4 cup chopped cucumber

•1/4 cup chopped cherry tomatoes

•1/4 cup chopped kalamata olives

•1/4 cup chopped almonds

•1/4 cup lemon juice

•1/4 cup extra virgin olive oil

•Salt and pepper to taste

Preparation:

1. In a large salad bowl, combine the mixed greens, red onion, bell peppers, cucumber, cherry tomatoes, kalamata olives, and almonds.

2. In a separate small bowl, whisk together the lemon juice, olive oil, salt, and pepper to create the vinaigrette.

3. Pour the vinaigrette over the salad and toss to combine. Top with the grilled chicken breast and serve immediately.

Turkey Meatballs with Zucchini Noodles

Serving: One

Cooking Time: 15 minutes

Ingredients:

•1 oz turkey meatballs

•2 oz zucchini noodles (store-bought or homemade)

•1/4 cup marinara sauce

•1/4 cup cooked spinach

•1/4 cup cooked broccoli

•1/4 cup cooked bell peppers

•1/4 cup cooked onions

•Salt and pepper to taste

Preparation:

1. In a large bowl, heat the zucchini noodles according to package instructions or your homemade recipe.

2. In a small saucepan, heat the marinara sauce over low heat. Add the turkey meatballs and cook until heated through.

3. In a large serving bowl, combine the cooked noodles, spinach, broccoli, bell peppers, and onions.

4. Pour the marinara sauce over the noodles and vegetables, and toss to combine.

5. Top with the heated turkey meatballs and season with salt and pepper to taste.

Honey Sesame Chicken with Broccolini

Serving: One

Cooking Time: 15 minutes

Ingredients:
- 4 oz grilled chicken breast

- 2 cups broccolini
- 1/4 cup honey
- 1 tbsp sesame oil
- Salt and pepper to taste
- 1/4 cup chopped almonds

Preparation:

1. In a large skillet, heat the sesame oil over medium heat.

2. Add the broccolini and cook until tender. In a small bowl, mix the honey, salt, and pepper.

3. Drizzle the honey mixture over the broccolini and cook for an additional 2-3 minutes until the broccolini is slightly caramelized.

4. Serve the grilled chicken breast over the honey sesame broccolini and top with chopped almonds.

Salmon Avocado Lettuce Wraps

Serving: One

Cooking Time: 15 minutes

Ingredients:

- 4 oz grilled salmon
- 1 avocado
- 1 large lettuce leaf
- 1 tbsp cream cheese
- 1 tbsp mayonnaise
- Salt and pepper to taste

Preparation:

1. In a small bowl, mix the cream cheese, mayonnaise, salt, and pepper. Spread the mixture onto the lettuce leaf.

2. In a separate bowl, mash the avocado with a fork and add 1 tbsp of water to keep it moist. Spread the avocado mixture on top of the lettuce.

3. Place the grilled salmon on top of the avocado and wrap the lettuce securely.

Watermelon Poke Bowls

Serving: One
Cooking Time: 10 minutes

Ingredients:
- 1/2 cup cooked quinoa
- 1 cup diced watermelon
- 1/4 cup chopped strawberries
- 1/4 cup chopped blueberries
- 1/4 cup chopped kiwi
- 1/4 cup chopped cucumber
- 1/4 cup chopped mint leaves
- 1 tbsp lime juice

•1 tbsp honey

•Salt and pepper to taste

Preparation:

1. In a large bowl, combine the cooked quinoa, watermelon, strawberries, blueberries, kiwi, cucumber, and mint leaves.

2. In a separate small bowl, whisk together the lime juice, honey, salt, and pepper to create a dressing.

3. Pour the dressing over the quinoa and fruit mixture and toss to combine. Serve immediately.

Cilantro-Lime Shrimp Wraps

Serving: One

Cooking Time: 15 minutes

Ingredients:

•4 oz shrimp, peeled and deveined

•Salt and pepper to taste

•1 tbsp olive oil

•1/2 cup chopped cilantro

•1/4 cup chopped lime juice

•1/4 cup chopped red onion

•1/4 cup chopped bell peppers

•1/4 cup chopped avocado

•2 large lettuce leaves

Preparation:

1. In a large bowl, toss the shrimp with salt and pepper. In a large skillet, heat the olive oil over medium heat.

2. Add the shrimp and cook until pink and cooked through.

3. In a small bowl, mix the cilantro, lime juice, red onion, bell peppers, and avocado.
4. Spread the mixture onto the lettuce leaves and top with the cooked shrimp.

Grilled Nectarine and Burrata Salad

Serving: One
Cooking Time: 10 minutes

Ingredients:
- 1/2 cup mixed greens
- 1 nectarine, sliced
- 1/4 cup chopped walnuts
- 1/4 cup cooked burrata cheese
- 1/4 cup lemon juice
- 1/4 cup extra virgin olive oil
- Salt and pepper to taste

Preparation:

1. In a large salad bowl, combine the mixed greens, nectarine, walnuts, and burrata cheese.

2. In a separate small bowl, whisk together the lemon juice, olive oil, salt, and pepper to create the vinaigrette.

3. Pour the vinaigrette over the salad and toss to combine.

Vegetable Egg Scramble

Serving: One

Ingredients

- 4 large eggs
- 1/4 cup fat-free milk
- 1/2 cup chopped green pepper
- 1/4 cup sliced green onions

•Salt and pepper to taste

Instructions:

1. In a bowl, lightly beat the eggs and mix in the fat-free milk.

2. Add the chopped green pepper and sliced green onions to the egg mixture.

3. Season with salt and pepper to taste.

4. Pour the egg mixture into a medium-heat nonstick skillet.

5. Cook, stirring constantly, until the eggs set. Serve immediately.

CHAPTER FOUR

DINNER RECIPES

Zucchini Lasagna

Serving: One

Cooking Time: 45 minutes

Ingredients:

- 1 medium zucchini, sliced lengthwise
- 1/2 cup marinara sauce
- 1/2 cup ricotta cheese
- 1/4 cup shredded mozzarella cheese
- 1/4 cup grated Parmesan cheese
- 1/2 teaspoon dried oregano

Instructions:

1. Preheat the oven to 375°F.

2. In a small baking dish, spread a thin layer of marinara sauce.

3. Place a layer of zucchini slices on top of the sauce.

4. Spread half of the ricotta cheese on the zucchini, then sprinkle with half of the mozzarella and Parmesan cheese.

5. Repeat the layers, ending with the remaining marinara sauce on top.

6. Sprinkle the top with dried oregano.

7. After baking for 30 minutes, cover the dish with foil. When the cheese is bubbling and brown, remove the foil and bake for a further 15 minutes.

Baked Salmon with Veggies and Quinoa

Serving: One

Cooking Time: 30 minutes

Ingredients:

•4 oz salmon fillet

•1/2 cup mixed vegetables (e.g., bell peppers, zucchini, cherry tomatoes)

•1/4 cup cooked quinoa

•1 tablespoon olive oil

•1/2 teaspoon dried dill

•Salt and pepper to taste

Instructions:

1. Preheat the oven to 400°F.

2. Place the salmon fillet on a baking sheet and surround it with the mixed vegetables.

3. Drizzle the olive oil over the salmon and vegetables, then sprinkle with dried dill, salt, and pepper.

4. Salmon should be cooked through and vegetables should be soft after 15 to 20 minutes in the oven.

5. Serve the salmon and vegetables over the cooked quinoa.

Stuffed Peppers

Serving: One

Cooking Time: 45 minutes

Ingredients:

- 2 large bell peppers
- 1/2 cup cooked ground turkey or beef
- 1/4 cup cooked rice
- 1/4 cup chopped onion
- 1/4 cup chopped tomatoes

•1/4 cup shredded cheddar cheese

•1/2 teaspoon dried oregano

•Salt and pepper to taste

Instructions:

1. Preheat the oven to 375°F.

2. Slice off the bell peppers' tops, then take out the seeds and membranes.

3. In a bowl, mix the cooked meat, rice, onion, tomatoes, half of the cheese, oregano, salt, and pepper.

4. Stuff the bell peppers with the meat and rice mixture and place them in a baking dish.

5. Sprinkle the remaining cheese on top of the stuffed peppers.

6. After baking the dish for 25 minutes with the foil removed, bake it for a further 10 minutes, or until the cheese is bubbling and melted.

Chicken Enchiladas on Gluten-Free Tortillas

Serving: One

Cooking Time: 40 minutes

Ingredients:

•4 oz cooked chicken, shredded

•2 gluten-free tortillas

•1/2 cup enchilada sauce

•1/4 cup shredded cheddar cheese

•1/4 cup chopped green onions

•1/4 cup chopped cilantro

Instructions:

1. Preheat the oven to 375°F.

2. In a small baking dish, spread a thin layer of enchilada sauce.

3. Place half of the shredded chicken on each tortilla, then roll up the tortillas and place them seam-side down in the baking dish.

4. Pour the remaining enchilada sauce over the tortillas, then sprinkle with the shredded cheese.

5. Bake for 20-25 minutes until the cheese is melted and bubbly.

6. Sprinkle the chopped green onions and cilantro on top before serving.

Vegetable Stir-Fry with Beef over Rice

Serving: One
Cooking Time: 30 minutes

Ingredients:

•4 oz beef, sliced

•1/2 cup mixed vegetables (e.g., bell peppers, broccoli, snap peas)

•1/4 cup sliced onion

•1/4 cup gluten-free stir-fry sauce

•1/2 cup cooked rice

•1 tablespoon vegetable oil

Instructions:

1. In a wok or large skillet, heat the vegetable oil over high heat.

2. Add the sliced beef and stir-fry for 2-3 minutes until browned.

3. Add the mixed vegetables and sliced onion to the wok and stir-fry for an additional 3-4 minutes until the vegetables are tender-crisp.

4. Pour the stir-fry sauce over the beef and vegetables and stir to combine.

5. Serve the stir-fry over the cooked rice.

Baked Cod with Lemon and Herbs

Serving: One

Cooking Time: 20 minutes

Ingredients:

•4 oz cod fillet

•1 tablespoon olive oil

•1/2 tablespoon fresh lemon juice

•1/2 teaspoon dried dill

•1/2 teaspoon dried thyme

•Salt and pepper to taste

Instructions:

1. Preheat the oven to 400°F.

2. Place the cod fillet on a baking sheet.

3. Drizzle the olive oil and lemon juice over the cod, then sprinkle with dried dill, thyme, salt, and pepper.

4. Bake for 15-20 minutes until the cod is cooked through and flakes easily with a fork.

Burgers with Gluten-Free Buns

Serving: One

Cooking Time: 20 minutes

Ingredients:

•4 oz ground beef or turkey

•1 gluten-free hamburger bun

•1/4 cup lettuce

•1/4 cup sliced tomato

•1/4 cup sliced red onion

•1 slice of cheese (optional)

•Salt and pepper to taste

Instructions:

1. Preheat a grill or grill pan over medium-high heat.

2. Season the ground meat with salt and pepper, then form it into a patty.

3. Grill the patty for 3-4 minutes on each side until it reaches your desired level of doneness.

4. Toast the gluten-free bun on the grill for 1-2 minutes.

5. Assemble the burger with the patty, lettuce, tomato, onion, and cheese (if using).

Gluten-Free Chicken Alfredo

Serving: One

Cooking Time: 25 minutes

Ingredients:

•4 oz cooked chicken, sliced

•1/2 cup gluten-free fettuccine

•1/2 cup broccoli florets

•1/2 cup cauliflower florets

•1/2 cup heavy cream

•1/4 cup grated Parmesan cheese

•1 tablespoon butter

•1 clove garlic, minced

•Salt and pepper to taste

Instructions:

1. Cook the gluten-free fettuccine according to the package instructions, adding the broccoli and cauliflower to the pot during the last 3 minutes of cooking.

2. Heat a large skillet over medium heat to melt the butter. Cook the minced garlic for one minute after adding it.

3. After adding the heavy cream, boil the mixture.

4. Once the sauce is smooth and creamy, stir in the grated Parmesan cheese.

5. Toss to coat in sauce after adding the cooked chicken, fettuccine, and veggies to the skillet.

6. Before serving, add salt and pepper to taste.

CHAPTER FIVE

SIDE RECIPES

Roasted Brussels Sprouts

Serving: One

Cooking Time: 25 minutes

Ingredients:

- 1 cup Brussels sprouts, trimmed and halved
- 1 tablespoon olive oil
- Salt and pepper to taste

Instructions:

1. Preheat the oven to 400°F.

2. Toss the Brussels sprouts with olive oil, salt, and pepper.

3. Spread the Brussels sprouts in a single layer on a baking sheet.

4. Roast for 20-25 minutes until the Brussels sprouts are tender and browned.

Garlic Lime Steamed Asparagus

Serving: One
Cooking Time: 10 minutes

Ingredients:
- 1/2 cup asparagus spears
- 1 clove garlic, minced
- 1 tablespoon fresh lime juice
- 1 tablespoon olive oil
- Salt and pepper to taste

Instructions:

1. In a steamer basket, steam the asparagus for 5-7 minutes until tender.

2. In a small bowl, whisk together the garlic, lime juice, olive oil, salt, and pepper.

3. Drizzle the garlic lime sauce over the steamed asparagus before serving.

Greek Chickpea Salad

Serving: One
Cooking Time: 10 minutes

Ingredients:
•1/2 cup canned chickpeas, drained and rinsed
•1/4 cup chopped cucumber
•1/4 cup chopped cherry tomatoes
•1/4 cup crumbled feta cheese
•1/4 cup chopped red onion
•1 tablespoon olive oil
•1 tablespoon fresh lemon juice
•Salt and pepper to taste

Instructions:

1. In a bowl, mix the chickpeas, cucumber, cherry tomatoes, feta cheese, and red onion.

2. In a small bowl, whisk together the olive oil, lemon juice, salt, and pepper to create the dressing.

3. Pour the dressing over the chickpea salad and toss to combine.

Mashed Sweet Potatoes with Maple Glaze

Serving: One

Cooking Time: 30 minutes

Ingredients:

- 1 medium sweet potato, peeled and cubed
- 1 tablespoon butter

•1 tablespoon maple syrup

•Salt and pepper to taste

Instructions:

1. Boil the sweet potato cubes in a pot of water for 15-20 minutes until tender.

2. Drain the sweet potatoes and mash them with the butter, maple syrup, salt, and pepper until smooth.

Cauliflower Gratin

Serving: One

Cooking Time: 45 minutes

Ingredients:

•1 cup cauliflower florets

•1/4 cup heavy cream

•1/4 cup grated Parmesan cheese

•1/4 teaspoon dried thyme

•Salt and pepper to taste

Instructions:

1. Preheat the oven to 375°F.

2. Steam the cauliflower florets for 5-7 minutes until tender.

3. In a small bowl, whisk together the heavy cream, Parmesan cheese, dried thyme, salt, and pepper.

4. Place the steamed cauliflower in a small baking dish and pour the cream mixture over it.

5. Bake for 20-25 minutes until the top is golden brown and bubbly.

Baked Wild Rice with Veggies

Serving: One

Cooking Time: 60 minutes

Ingredients:

- 1/4 cup wild rice
- 1/2 cup mixed vegetables (e.g., bell peppers, carrots, peas)
- 1/2 cup vegetable broth
- 1 tablespoon olive oil
- Salt and pepper to taste

Instructions:

1. Preheat the oven to 375°F.

2. In a small baking dish, combine the wild rice, mixed vegetables, vegetable broth, olive oil, salt, and pepper.

3. Cover the dish with foil and bake for 45-50 minutes until the rice is tender and the liquid is absorbed.

Sauteed Green Beans with Garlic

Serving: One
Cooking Time: 15 minutes

Ingredients:
- 1/2 cup green beans, trimmed
- 1 clove garlic, minced
- 1 tablespoon olive oil
- Salt and pepper to taste

Instructions:

1. In a skillet, heat the olive oil over medium heat.

2. Add the green beans and garlic to the skillet and sauté for 8-10 minutes until the green beans are tender-crisp.

3. Season with salt and pepper to taste before serving.

Oven Roasted Parmesan Asparagus

Serving: One

Cooking Time: 15 minutes

Ingredients:

- 1/2 cup asparagus spears
- 1 tablespoon olive oil
- 2 tablespoons grated Parmesan cheese
- Salt and pepper to taste

Instructions:

1. Preheat the oven to 400°F.

2. Toss the asparagus with olive oil, salt, and pepper.

3. Spread the asparagus in a single layer on a baking sheet.

4. Roast for 10-12 minutes until the asparagus is tender.

5. Sprinkle the grated Parmesan cheese over the asparagus and return to the oven for 2-3 minutes until the cheese is melted and bubbly.

Mushy Peas

Serving: One
Cooking Time: 15 minutes

Ingredients:

- 1/2 cup frozen peas
- 1 tablespoon butter
- Salt and pepper to taste

Instructions:

1. In a small saucepan, melt the butter over medium heat.

2. Add the frozen peas to the saucepan and cook for 5-7 minutes until the peas are tender.

3. Mash the peas with a fork until they reach your desired consistency.

4. Season with salt and pepper to taste before serving.

CHAPTER SIX

SNACK RECIPES

Hummus with Rice Crackers

Serving: One

Ingredients:
- 1/4 cup hummus
- 1 serving of gluten-free rice crackers

Instructions:

1. Place the hummus in a small bowl for dipping.

2. Serve with the gluten-free rice crackers.

Sunflower Seeds

Serving: One

Ingredients:
•1/4 cup sunflower seeds

Instructions:

1. Enjoy the sunflower seeds as a simple and nutritious snack.

Fresh Fruit

Serving: One

Ingredients:
•1 serving of your favorite fresh fruit (e.g., apple, banana, orange)

Instructions:

1. Wash and prepare the fruit as needed.

2. Enjoy the fresh fruit as a healthy snack.

String Cheese

Serving: One

Ingredients:

- 1 stick of gluten-free string cheese

Instructions:

1. Simply unwrap and enjoy the string cheese as a convenient and satisfying snack.

Raisins

Serving: One

Ingredients:

•1/4 cup raisins

Instructions:

1. Enjoy the raisins as a naturally sweet and portable snack.

Popcorn with Dark Chocolate and Dried Fruit

Serving: One

Ingredients:

•1/4 cup popcorn kernels

•1/4 cup dark chocolate chips

•1/4 cup dried fruit (e.g., cranberries, raisins, cherries)

Instructions:

1. Pop the popcorn kernels according to the package instructions.

2. Melt the dark chocolate chips in the microwave or on the stovetop.

3. Drizzle the melted chocolate over the popcorn and sprinkle with the dried fruit.

Gluten-Free Energy Balls

Serving: One

Ingredients:
- 1/2 cup gluten-free rolled oats
- 1/4 cup almond butter
- 1/4 cup honey
- 1/4 cup shredded coconut
- 1/4 cup mini chocolate chips

Instructions:

Instructions:

1. In a bowl, mix the rolled oats, almond butter, and honey until well combined.

2. Stir in the shredded coconut and mini chocolate chips.

3. Roll the mixture into small balls and refrigerate until firm.

Sweet Potato Chips with Tzatziki Sauce

Serving: One
Cooking Time: 30 minutes

Ingredients:
•1 medium sweet potato, peeled and sliced into thin rounds
•1 tablespoon olive oil

•Salt and pepper to taste

•1/2 cup plain Greek yogurt

•1/4 cup grated cucumber

•1 clove garlic, minced

•1 tablespoon chopped fresh dill

•1 tablespoon fresh lemon juice

Instructions:

1. Preheat the oven to 400°F.

2. Toss the sweet potato rounds with olive oil, salt, and pepper.

3. Spread the sweet potato rounds in a single layer on a baking sheet.

4. Bake for 20-25 minutes until the sweet potato chips are crispy and golden brown.

5. While the sweet potato chips are baking, prepare the tzatziki sauce by mixing the Greek yogurt, grated cucumber, minced garlic, chopped fresh dill, and fresh lemon juice in a small bowl.

6. Serve the sweet potato chips with the tzatziki sauce for dipping.

CHAPTER SEVEN

SOUP & STEW RECIPES

Cabbage and White Bean Stew

Serving: One

Cooking Time: 30 minutes

Ingredients:

- 1/2 cup white beans, cooked
- 1 cup chopped cabbage
- 1/4 cup chopped onion
- 1 clove garlic, minced
- 1/2 cup gluten-free vegetable broth
- 1/2 teaspoon dried thyme
- Salt and pepper to taste

Instructions:

1. In a pot, sauté the onion and garlic until softened.

2. Add the cabbage, white beans, vegetable broth, thyme, salt, and pepper.

3. Simmer for 20 minutes until the cabbage is tender.

Cream of Mushroom Soup

Serving: One
Cooking Time: 30 minutes

Ingredients:
- 1 cup sliced mushrooms
- 1/4 cup chopped onion
- 1 clove garlic, minced
- 1 tablespoon butter
- 1 tablespoon gluten-free all-purpose flour

•1 cup gluten-free chicken or vegetable broth

•1/2 cup milk

Instructions:

1. In a pot, sauté the mushrooms, onion, and garlic in butter until softened.

2. Stir in the gluten-free flour and cook for 1 minute.

3. Gradually stir in the broth and milk.

4. Simmer for 10 minutes until thickened.

Lentil and Sausage Stew

Serving: One

Cooking Time: 45 minutes

Ingredients:

- 1/2 cup cooked lentils
- 1/4 cup chopped onion
- 1/4 cup chopped carrot
- 1/4 cup chopped celery
- 1/2 cup gluten-free chicken or vegetable broth
- 1 cooked gluten-free sausage, sliced
- 1/2 teaspoon dried thyme
- Salt and pepper to taste

Instructions:

1. In a pot, sauté the onion, carrot, and celery until softened.

2. Add the lentils, broth, sausage, thyme, salt, and pepper.

3. Simmer for 30 minutes until the flavors are blended.

Roasted Acorn Squash Soup

Serving: One

Cooking Time: 1 hour

Ingredients:

- 1 acorn squash, halved and seeded
- 1 tablespoon olive oil
- 1/4 cup chopped onion
- 1 clove garlic, minced
- 1/2 teaspoon ground cumin
- 1/4 teaspoon ground cinnamon
- 2 cups gluten-free chicken or vegetable broth
- Salt and pepper to taste

Instructions:

1. Preheat the oven to 400°F.

2. Place the acorn squash, cut side down, on a baking sheet.

3. Roast for 45 minutes until tender.

4. In a pot, sauté the onion and garlic in olive oil until softened.

5. Scoop the flesh of the acorn squash into the pot.

7. Stir in the cumin, cinnamon, and broth.

8. Simmer for 10 minutes.

9. Purée the soup until smooth.

Chicken Tortilla Soup

Serving: One
Cooking Time: 30 minutes

Ingredients:

- 1/2 cup cooked chicken, shredded
- 1/4 cup chopped onion
- 1/4 cup chopped bell pepper
- 1 clove garlic, minced
- 1/2 teaspoon ground cumin
- 1/4 teaspoon chili powder
- 2 cups gluten-free chicken broth
- 1/4 cup crushed gluten-free tortilla chips

Instructions:

1. In a pot, sauté the onion, bell pepper, and garlic until softened.

2. Stir in the cumin, chili powder, and broth.

Simmer for 15 minutes.

3. Stir in the chicken and tortilla chips.

4. Simmer for 5 minutes.

Creamy Carrot Ginger Soup

Serving: One

Cooking Time: 30 minutes

Ingredients:
- 1 cup chopped carrots
- 1/4 cup chopped onion
- 1 clove garlic, minced
- 1/2 tablespoon grated fresh ginger
- 1 cup gluten-free vegetable broth
- 1/4 cup coconut milk
- Salt and pepper to taste

Instructions:

1. In a pot, sauté the onion, garlic, and ginger until softened.

2. Add the carrots and broth, and simmer for 20 minutes until the carrots are tender.
3. Purée the soup until smooth, and stir in the coconut milk.

Split Pea Soup

Serving: One
Cooking Time: 1 hour

Ingredients:
- 1/2 cup dried split peas
- 1/4 cup chopped onion
- 1/4 cup chopped carrot
- 1/4 cup chopped celery
- 2 cups gluten-free vegetable broth
- 1 cooked gluten-free ham hock, chopped

•Salt and pepper to taste

Instructions:

1. In a pot, sauté the onion, carrot, and celery until softened.

2. Add the split peas, broth, and ham hock, and simmer for 45 minutes until the peas are tender.

Vegetable Beef Soup

Serving: One
Cooking Time: 1 hour

Ingredients:
•4 oz beef, cubed
•1/4 cup chopped onion
•1/4 cup chopped carrot
•1/4 cup chopped celery
•2 cups gluten-free beef broth

•1/2 cup chopped tomatoes

•Salt and pepper to taste

Instructions:

1. In a pot, sauté the beef, onion, carrot, and celery until the beef is browned.
2. Add the broth and tomatoes, and simmer for 45 minutes until the beef is tender.

CHAPTER EIGHT

FISH & SEAFOOD RECIPES

Shrimp, Peas & Pasta

Serving: One

Cooking Time: 15 minutes

Ingredients:

•4 oz shrimp, peeled and deveined

•1/2 cup frozen peas

•4 oz gluten-free pasta

•1 tablespoon olive oil

•Salt and pepper to taste

Instructions:

1. Cook the pasta according to package

instructions.

2. Heat the olive oil in a big skillet over medium heat.

3 Cook the prawns for 2-3 minutes on each side, or until they are cooked through and pink.

4. Add the peas and cook for 1 minute until heated through.

5. Drain the pasta and serve topped with the shrimp and peas.

Thrifty Thursday Salmon

Serving: One
Cooking Time: 15 minutes

Ingredients:
•4 oz salmon fillet
•1 tablespoon olive oil

•Salt and pepper to taste

Instructions:

1. Preheat the oven to 400°F.

2. In an oven-safe skillet, heat the olive oil over medium heat.

3. Place the salmon fillet in the skillet, skin-side down, and cook for 2 minutes until the skin is crispy.

4. Carefully flip the salmon and cook for another 2 minutes until cooked through.

5. Season with salt and pepper to taste.

Fish Tacos with Creamy Salsa

Serving: One

Cooking Time: 15 minutes

Ingredients:

•4 oz cod fillet

•1 tablespoon olive oil

•1/2 cup gluten-free tortilla chips

•1/2 cup salsa

•1/2 cup Greek yogurt

•Salt and pepper to taste

Instructions:

1. In a skillet, heat the olive oil over medium heat.

2. Place the cod fillet in the skillet and cook for 2-3 minutes per side until cooked through.

3. Warm the gluten-free tortilla chips in a dry skillet or directly over the stove.

4. Assemble the tacos with the cooked cod, salsa, and Greek yogurt.

Seafood Chowder

Serving: One
Cooking Time: 20 minutes

Ingredients:
- 1 tablespoon olive oil
- 1/2 cup chopped onion
- 1/2 cup chopped carrot
- 1/2 cup chopped celery
- 2 cups gluten-free fish or seafood broth
- 1/2 cup white wine or dry sherry
- 1/4 cup gluten-free flour
- Salt and pepper to taste
- 1 cup mixed seafood (e.g., fish, shellfish, and/or shrimp)

Instructions:

1. In a large pot, heat the olive oil over medium heat.

2. Sauté the onion, carrot, and celery until softened.

3. Add the broth, wine, and flour, and cook for 5 minutes, stirring constantly, to create a roux.

4. Bring the soup to a boil, then reduce the heat and simmer for 10 minutes.

5. Add the seafood and cook for an additional 5 minutes until the seafood is cooked through.

6. Season with salt and pepper to taste.

Baked White Fish with Roasted Potatoes

Serving: One
Cooking Time: 20 minutes

Ingredients:

•4 oz white fish fillet (e.g., cod, tilapia, or halibut)

•1 tablespoon olive oil

•Salt and pepper to taste

•1 cup chopped potatoes

•1 tablespoon olive oil

•Salt and pepper to taste

Instructions:

1. Preheat the oven to 400°F.

2. In a baking dish, drizzle 1 tablespoon of olive oil. Place the fish fillet in the dish and season with salt and pepper to taste.

3. In a separate bowl, toss the chopped potatoes with 1 tablespoon of olive oil, salt, and pepper.

4. Roast the fish and potatoes in the preheated oven for 15-20 minutes until the fish flakes easily with a fork and the potatoes are tender.

Balsamic Glazed Salmon

Serving: One
Cooking Time: 15 minutes

Ingredients:
- 4 oz salmon filet
- 1 tablespoon olive oil
- 2 tablespoons balsamic vinegar
- 1 tablespoon honey
- Salt and pepper to taste

Instructions:

1. Preheat the oven to 400°F.

2. In a small bowl, mix the balsamic vinegar, honey, and salt and pepper.

3. In a skillet, heat the olive oil over medium heat.

4. Place the salmon fillet in the skillet and cook for 2-3 minutes per side until cooked through.

5. Drizzle the glaze over the cooked salmon and serve.

Grilled Halibut with Mango Salsa

Serving: One

Cooking Time: 20 minutes

Ingredients:

- 1 halibut filet
- 1 tablespoon olive oil
- Salt and pepper to taste
- 1 large ripe mango, diced
- 1/4 cup red onion, finely chopped
- 1/4 cup fresh cilantro, chopped
- 1 jalapeño, seeded and finely chopped
- 2 tablespoons fresh lime juice

Instructions:

1. Preheat the grill to medium-high heat.

2. Brush the halibut fillet with olive oil and season with salt and pepper.

3. Grill the halibut for 4-5 minutes per side until it is cooked through and has grill marks.

4. In a bowl, combine the diced mango, red onion, cilantro, jalapeño, and lime juice to make the salsa.

5. Serve the grilled halibut with the mango salsa on top.

Roasted Salmon with Corn Relish

Serving: One

Cooking Time: 30 minutes

Ingredients:
- 1 salmon fillet

•1 tablespoon olive oil

•Salt and pepper to taste

•1 cup corn kernels

•1/4 cup diced red bell pepper

•2 tablespoons chopped fresh cilantro

•1 tablespoon lime juice

•1/2 teaspoon cumin

•1/4 teaspoon chili powder

Instructions:

1. Preheat the oven to 400°F.

2. Place the salmon fillet on a baking sheet and drizzle with olive oil. Season with salt and pepper.

3. In a bowl, mix the corn, red bell pepper, cilantro, lime juice, cumin, and chili powder to make the relish.

4. Spoon the relish over the salmon.

5. Roast for 15-20 minutes until the salmon is cooked through and the relish is slightly charred.

CHAPTER NINE

DESSERT RECIPES

Cheesecake Stuffed Strawberries

Serving: One

Cooking Time: 15 minutes

Ingredients:

- 4 large strawberries
- 2 oz cream cheese, softened
- 1 tablespoon powdered sugar
- 1/4 teaspoon vanilla extract

Instructions:

1. Cut off the tops of the strawberries and scoop out the centers with a small spoon.

2. In a bowl, mix the cream cheese, powdered sugar, and vanilla extract.

3. Spoon the cream cheese mixture into the hollowed-out strawberries. Serve chilled.

Coconut-Pecan Tart

Serving: One
Cooking Time: 30 minutes

Ingredients:
- 1/4 cup coconut flour
- 1/4 cup almond flour
- 1/4 cup chopped pecans
- 2 tablespoons coconut oil, melted

•2 tablespoons honey

•1/4 teaspoon salt

Instructions:

1. Preheat the oven to 350°F.

2. In a bowl, mix the coconut flour, almond flour, chopped pecans, coconut oil, honey, and salt.

3. Press the mixture into a small tart pan.

4. Bake for 15-20 minutes until golden brown.

Let cool before serving.

Flourless Chocolate Avocado Brownies

Serving: One

Cooking Time: 30 minutes

Ingredients:

•1 ripe avocado

•1/2 cup cocoa powder

•1/2 cup honey

•1 egg

•1/2 teaspoon baking soda

•1/4 teaspoon salt

Instructions:

1. Preheat the oven to 350°F.

2. Puree the avocado in a blender or food processor until it's smooth.

3. Blend well after adding the cocoa powder, honey, egg, baking soda, and salt.

4. Fill a baking dish with oil before pouring the batter in.

5. A toothpick inserted in the center should come out clean after baking for 20 to 25 minutes.

6. Let cool before serving.

Strawberry-Lemonade Angel Pie

Serving: One
Cooking Time: 30 minutes

Ingredients:
- 1 gluten-free graham cracker crust
- 1/2 cup fresh lemon juice
- 1/2 cup sugar
- 1/4 cup cornstarch
- 1/4 teaspoon salt
- 1/2 cup water
- 1/2 cup chopped fresh strawberries

•1/2 cup whipped cream

Instructions:

1. In a saucepan, whisk together the lemon juice, sugar, cornstarch, salt, and water.

2. Cook over medium heat, stirring constantly, until the mixture thickens and boils.

3. Remove from heat and stir in the chopped strawberries.

4. Pour the mixture into the graham cracker crust and let cool.

5. Top with whipped cream before serving.

Vegan Blueberry Crisp

Serving: One

Cooking Time: 30 minutes

Ingredients:

- 1/2 cup gluten-free rolled oats
- 1/4 cup almond flour
- 1/4 cup chopped pecans
- 2 tablespoons coconut oil, melted
- 2 tablespoons maple syrup
- 1/4 teaspoon cinnamon
- 1 cup fresh blueberries

Instructions:

1. Preheat the oven to 350°F.

2. In a bowl, mix the rolled oats, almond flour, chopped pecans, coconut oil, maple syrup, and cinnamon.

3. Spread the blueberries in a small baking dish.

4. Sprinkle the oat mixture over the blueberries.

5. Bake for 20-25 minutes until the topping is golden brown and the blueberries are bubbling.

6. Let cool before serving.

Soft and Chewy Gluten-free Ginger Snaps

Serving: One
Cooking Time: 20 minutes

Ingredients:
- 1/2 cup almond flour
- 1/2 cup gluten-free all-purpose flour
- 1/4 cup coconut sugar

•1/4 cup molasses

•1/4 cup coconut oil, melted

•1 egg

•1 teaspoon ground ginger

•1/2 teaspoon ground cinnamon

•1/4 teaspoon ground cloves

•1/4 teaspoon salt

Instructions:

1. Preheat the oven to 350°F.

2. In a bowl, mix the almond flour, gluten-free all-purpose flour, coconut sugar, molasses, coconut oil, egg, ginger, cinnamon, cloves, and salt.

3. Roll the dough into small balls and place them on a baking sheet.

4. Bake for 10-12 minutes until the cookies are set and slightly golden.

5. Let cool before serving.

Tasty Gluten-Free Apple Crisp

Serving: One

Cooking Time: 30 minutes

Ingredients:

•1 apple, peeled and sliced

•1/4 cup gluten-free rolled oats

•1/4 cup almond flour

•2 tablespoons coconut sugar

•2 tablespoons coconut oil, melted

•1/4 teaspoon cinnamon

•1/4 teaspoon salt

Instructions:

1. Preheat the oven to 350°F.

2. Spread the sliced apple in a small baking dish.

3. In a bowl, mix the rolled oats, almond flour, coconut sugar, coconut oil, cinnamon, and salt.

4. Sprinkle the oat mixture over the apples.

5. Bake for 20-25 minutes until the topping is golden brown and the apples are tender.

6. Let cool before serving.

Fudgy Sweet Potato Brownies

Serving: One

Cooking Time: 30 minutes

Ingredients:

- 1/2 cup mashed sweet potato
- 1/2 cup almond flour

•1/4 cup cocoa powder

•1/4 cup honey

•1 egg

•1/2 teaspoon baking soda

•1/4 teaspoon salt

Instructions:

1. Preheat the oven to 350°F.

2. In a bowl, mix the mashed sweet potato, almond flour, cocoa powder, honey, egg, baking soda, and salt.

3. Pour the batter into a greased baking dish.

4. Bake for 20-25 minutes until a toothpick inserted into the center comes out clean.

5. Let cool before serving.

7-DAY MEAL PLAN

Day 1

Breakfast: Banana Oat Pancakes

Lunch: Chicken, Bean, & Spinach Stew

Dinner: Zucchini Lasagna

Snack: Hummus with Rice Crackers

Day 2

Breakfast: Rhubarb Muffins

Lunch: Grilled Chicken over Greens Lemon Vinaigrette

Dinner: Baked Salmon with Veggies and Quinoa

Snack: Fresh Fruit

Day 3

Breakfast: Cinnamon Quinoa Bake

Lunch: Turkey Meatballs with Zucchini Noodles

Dinner: Stuffed Peppers

Snack: Sunflower Seeds

Day 4

Breakfast: Nutty Millet Breakfast Bowl

Lunch: Watermelon Poke Bowls

Dinner: Chicken Enchiladas on Gluten-Free Tortillas

Snack: String Cheese

Day 5

Breakfast: Tomato Tart

Lunch: Honey Sesame Chicken with Broccolini

Dinner: Vegetable Stir-Fry with Beef over Rice

Snack: Popcorn with Dark Chocolate and Dried Fruit

Day 6

Breakfast: Gluten-Free Pancakes

Lunch: Salmon Avocado Lettuce Wraps

Dinner: Baked Cod with Lemon and Herbs

Snack: Sweet Potato Chips with Tzatziki Sauce

Day 7

Breakfast: Creamy Polenta with Chorizo

Lunch: Grilled Nectarine and Burrata Salad

Dinner: Burgers with Gluten-Free Buns

Snack: Fresh Fruit

Feel free to adjust the plan based on personal preferences and dietary needs!

CONCLUSION

In concluding this Celiac Disease Cookbook for Seniors, our culinary journey has been a celebration of flavor, nourishment, and well-being. Each recipe is a testament to the belief that a gluten-free lifestyle can be both delectable and health-enhancing. As seniors embark on this gastronomic adventure, they not only embrace a diet tailored to manage Celiac Disease but also indulge in a symphony of tastes that elevate every meal.

From the comforting embrace of Banana Oat Pancakes to the savory delights of Zucchini Lasagna and the sweet endings of Fudgy Sweet Potato Brownies, this cookbook transcends the boundaries of dietary restrictions.

It empowers seniors to savor each bite with the knowledge that they are nourishing their bodies and fostering digestive health.

Remember, this isn't just about eliminating gluten; it's a holistic approach to enjoying life through mindful eating. The carefully crafted meal plans, diverse recipes, and nutritional insights are designed to support seniors on their journey to improved health and vitality. By adopting this gluten-free lifestyle, readers aren't just managing Celiac Disease; they're cultivating a relationship with food that prioritizes wellness.

As you embrace the recipes within these pages, envision a life where each meal is a joyful experience, a moment to cherish. Let this cookbook be your guide to a fulfilling and vibrant chapter, free from the constraints of Celiac-related concerns. Your health is an invaluable treasure, and through these recipes, you have the tools to nurture it.

So, dear reader, take charge of your well-being. Let this cookbook be the catalyst for a renewed relationship with food, a journey where every dish becomes a celebration of life and health. Bon appétit!

www.ingramcontent.com/pod-product-compliance
Lightning Source LLC
Chambersburg PA
CBHW070855260726

48661CB00004B/1424